S0-AFX-744

Make Your Own Beauty Masks

38 Simple, All-Natural
Recipes for Healthy Skin

New York

How to Use This Book

Use the ten sheet masks included in the front envelope to keep nutrients in and dirt out, or apply the mask mixtures directly to your face for maximum refreshment.

Your Key to Beauty

Look for these icons on each recipe to find the perfect mask for you.

	Healing
	Plumping
	Hydrating
	Smoothing
	Brightening
	Acne-fighting
	Pore-shrinking
	Oil-eliminating
	Breakout-busting
	Redness-reducing

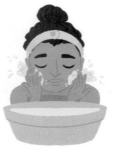

Pre-Mask Prep

Wash your face and neck with warm water and an oil-free cleanser to open up your pores.

OPTIONAL: You may also want to use a toner.

Applying Your Mask

If you're skipping the sheet mask, evenly apply the mixture directly to your face in an upward motion using your fingers or a facial brush.

If you're using a sheet mask, remove one sheet from the envelope located at the front of this book. Then do one of the following:

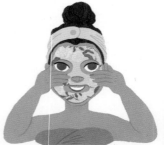
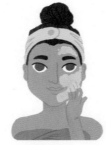

OPTION 1: Apply the mixture directly to your skin, and then place the sheet mask on top.

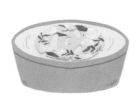
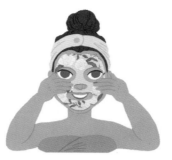
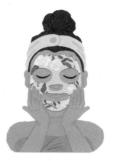

OPTION 2: Soak the sheet mask in the mixture for a minute or two. Once the sheet is thoroughly soaked, hold it above the mixture and let any excess liquid drop off. You don't want the mask so wet that it falls right off! Then gently place it over your face.

BABY STEPS: Always test your mask mixture on the back of your hand or wrist *before* applying it to your face to see how your skin reacts.

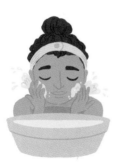
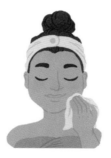
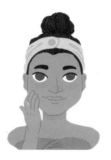

Post-Mask Care

Remove your mask after 10–20 minutes. Splash your face with lukewarm water to rinse away any excess mask mixture, then follow with cool water to close your pores. Gently pat your skin dry with a clean towel.

Preserving Your Masks

Your mask mixtures can remain in airtight containers in the refrigerator for three days. After that, toss 'em! Your sheet masks, however, are single-use—one-and-done only.

Measurement Conversion Chart

1 teaspoon ≈ 5 mL

1 tablespoon ≈ 15 mL

¼ cup ≈ 60 mL

⅓ cup ≈ 80 mL

½ cup ≈ 120 mL

1 cup ≈ 240 mL

MASK CONTENTS

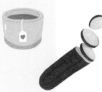

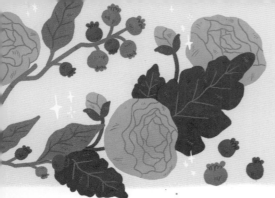

Your Berry Best

Think of this mask as your deliciously blue fountain of youth. Blueberries are bursting with antioxidants and vitamin C to pump up collagen and keep skin firm.

INGREDIENTS

 2 tablespoons plain Greek yogurt

8–10 blueberries (thawed if frozen)

2 teaspoons raw honey

TOOLS

 Blender

Plumping
Smoothing
Brightening
Redness-reducing

 1 Put all ingredients into the blender.

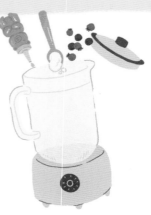

 2 Blend until the mixture is smooth.

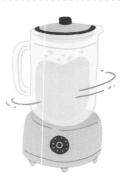

3 Apply for 10–20 minutes, then rinse.

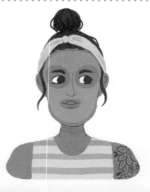

An Appeeling Look

Stop monkeying around and nourish your skin with banana, turmeric, and baking soda to naturally cleanse, smooth, and brighten.

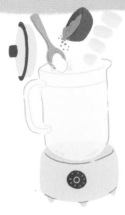

1   Put all ingredients into the blender.

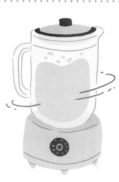

2   Blend until the mixture is smooth.

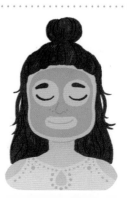

3   Apply for 10–20 minutes, then rinse.

INGREDIENTS

 1 banana

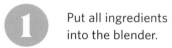 ½ teaspoon baking soda

 ½ teaspoon ground turmeric

TOOLS

 Blender

First time using baking soda for skincare? Test this mixture on the inside of your wrist beforehand.

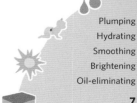

Plumping
Hydrating
Smoothing
Brightening
Oil-eliminating

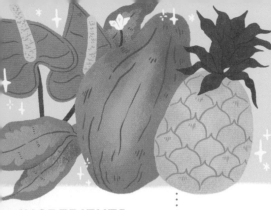

Tropic Like It's Hot

Treat your skin to an island vacation. This papaya-and-pineapple remedy removes dry skin, moisturizes, and minimizes pores. You'll never want to go back to the mainland.

INGREDIENTS

 ½ of one papaya (skin peeled, seeds removed, cut into pieces, thawed if frozen)

 1 cup pineapple (cut into pieces, thawed if frozen)

 1 tablespoon raw honey

TOOLS

 Blender

Hydrating
Smoothing
Brightening
Pore-shrinking
Breakout-busting

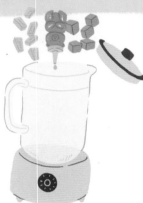

 1 Put all ingredients into the blender.

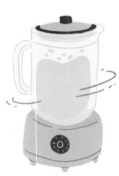 **2** Blend until the mixture is smooth.

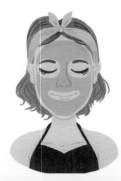 **3** Apply for 10–20 minutes, then rinse.

Do You Like Piña Coladas?

Sit back and relax as this poolside potion reduces skin-damaging free radicals, lightens dark spots and blemishes, and firms and repairs your skin.

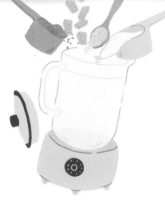

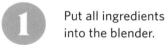

1 Put all ingredients into the blender.

INGREDIENTS

 ½ cup pineapple (cut into pieces, thawed if frozen)

 ½ cup coconut milk

 ¼ cup brown sugar

 1 tablespoon grated fresh or ground ginger

2 Blend until the mixture is smooth.

TOOLS

 Blender

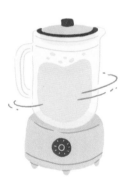

3 Apply for 10–20 minutes, then rinse.

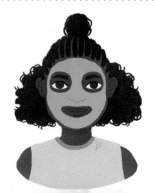

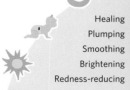

Healing
Plumping
Smoothing
Brightening
Redness-reducing

9

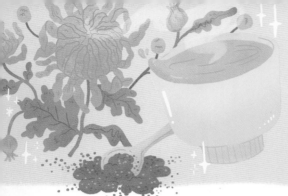

Mamma Chia!

Here we go again! This anti-inflammatory, omega-3-rich elixir reduces redness, restores moisture, and revives dull, flat-looking skin.

SKIP THE SHEET! This mask goes directly on your face!

INGREDIENTS

 4 tablespoons freshly brewed strong green tea

2 tablespoons chia seeds

3 teaspoons raw honey

TOOLS

Mixing bowl

Spoon

Healing
Plumping
Hydrating
Brightening
Redness-reducing

1 Brew the tea with one cup of water and let steep for 3 minutes. Allow the tea to cool slightly.

2 Put all ingredients into the mixing bowl.

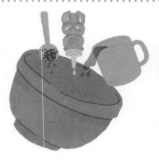

3 Mix into a smooth paste.

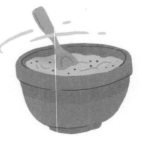

4 Apply for 10–20 minutes, then rinse.

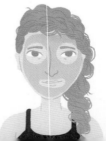

Honey, I Shrunk My Pores

You don't need Rick Moranis's ray gun to shrink your pores. A simple mixture of kefir and honey will bring those babies down to size while hydrating and moisturizing at the same time.

1 Put all ingredients into the mixing bowl.

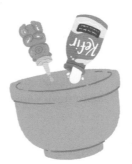

INGREDIENTS

 ⅓ cup plain kefir

 1 tablespoon raw honey

TOOLS

 Mixing bowl

Spoon

2 Mix until smooth.

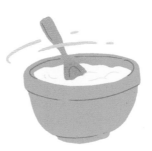

3 Apply for 10–20 minutes, then rinse.

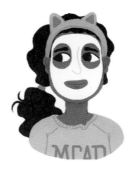

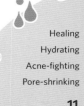

Healing
Hydrating
Acne-fighting
Pore-shrinking

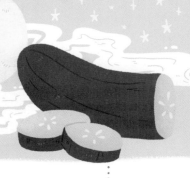

Cucumber Slumber

Hey, sleeping beauty! Slap this mask on before bedtime to keep calm and soothe on. It's cooling, calming, and oh-so cucumbery! Just remember to wash it off before falling asleep.

INGREDIENTS

 ½ of one cucumber (cut into slices)

 1 teaspoon baking soda

 1 teaspoon olive oil

TOOLS

 Blender

First time using baking soda for skincare? Test this mixture on the inside of your wrist beforehand.

Healing
Hydrating
Smoothing

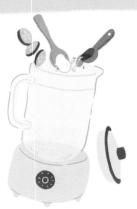

1 Put all ingredients into the blender.

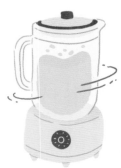

2 Blend until the mixture is smooth.

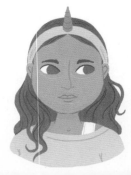

3 Apply for 10–20 minutes, then rinse.

Take Carrot Yourself

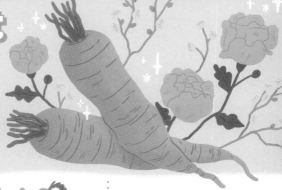

You've probably heard how good carrots are for your eyes. Well, the same can be said for your skin. The beta-carotene found in the bright orange roots smooths, protects, and firms.

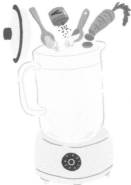

1 Put all ingredients into the blender.

INGREDIENTS

1 medium-size carrot (peeled and chopped)

2 teaspoons coconut milk

1 teaspoon room-temperature coconut oil

1 teaspoon ground cinnamon

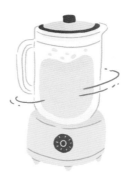

2 Blend until the mixture is smooth.

TOOLS

Blender

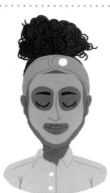

3 Apply for 10–20 minutes, then rinse.

FYI: Cinnamon might cause your skin to tingle. If this feeling isn't your thing, wash off this mask ASAP.

Healing
Plumping
Hydrating
Smoothing
Redness-reducing

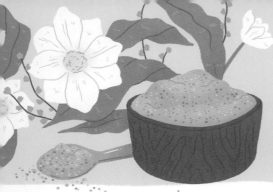

You're Too Sweet!

This sugary-sweet mix buffs away dry skin for an instantly brighter look!

SKIP THE SHEET! This mask goes directly on your face!

INGREDIENTS

 2 tablespoons brown sugar

 2 teaspoons room-temperature coconut oil

TOOLS

 Mixing bowl

 Spoon

Hydrating

Brightening

14

1 Put all ingredients into the mixing bowl.

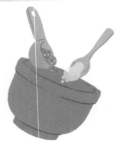

2 Mix into a smooth paste.

3 Apply for 10–20 minutes.

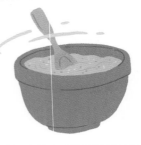

4 Gently massage your face with small, circular motions for 2 minutes, then rinse.

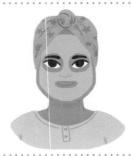

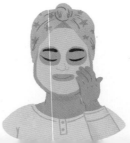

I'll Never Take You for Pomegranate

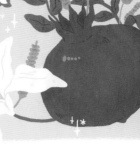

Your skin takes a beating throughout the day. Keep it elastic, energized, and glowing with the replenishing powers of pomegranate juice.

INGREDIENTS

 2 tablespoons plain Greek yogurt

 1 tablespoon raw honey

 1 tablespoon pomegranate juice

TOOLS

 Mixing bowl

 Spoon

 1 Put all ingredients into the mixing bowl.

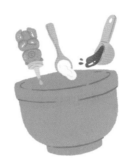

 2 Mix until smooth.

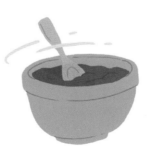

 3 Apply for 10–20 minutes, then rinse.

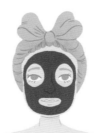

Plumping
Hydrating
Smoothing
Brightening
Redness-reducing

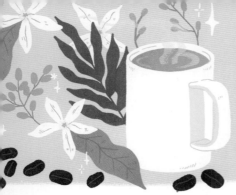

Extra-Grande Mocha Latte

Pick up some extra beans on your next coffee run! Caffeine tightens skin, making it look smooth and toned, while coffee grounds gently exfoliate, cleansing pores of grit and grime.

INGREDIENTS

 2 tablespoons coffee grounds

 2 tablespoons cocoa powder

 3 tablespoons plain Greek yogurt

 1 tablespoon raw honey

TOOLS

 Mixing bowl

 Spoon

Plumping
Smoothing
Oil-eliminating
Breakout-busting

1 Put all ingredients into the mixing bowl.

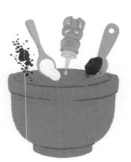

2 Mix into a smooth paste.

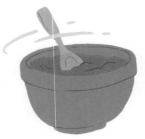

3 Apply for 10–20 minutes, then rinse.

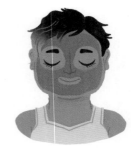

Pumpkin Spice See-Ya-Latte, Acne

It's PSL versus pimples! Your favorite fall combo is a natural anti-inflammatory that reduces oil and acne and clears pores. No matter the season, this mask is perfect for a cozy night in.

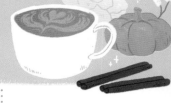

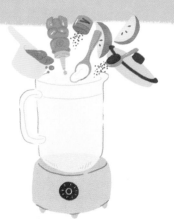

1 Put all ingredients into the blender.

2 Blend until the mixture is smooth.

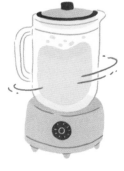

INGREDIENTS

 ½ cup pumpkin puree

 ½ of one apple (peeled, cored, and sliced)

 1 tablespoon raw honey

 1 tablespoon plain Greek yogurt

 1 teaspoon ground cinnamon

 1 teaspoon ground nutmeg

TOOLS

 Blender

3 Apply for 10–20 minutes, then rinse.

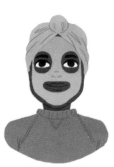

FYI: Nutmeg and cinnamon might cause your skin to tingle. If this feeling isn't your thing, wash off this mask ASAP.

Acne-fighting
Oil-eliminating
Breakout-busting

Face the Facts

COCONUT OIL is jam-packed with vitamin E, essential amino acids, and proteins that hydrate your skin. It also includes lauric and caprylic acids, which eat away at the nasty stuff that gloms on to your face throughout the day.

The omega-3 fatty acids found in **CHIA SEEDS** are a must-have for happy, healthy skin. These good fats reduce the production of inflammatory compounds and act as a barrier for pore protection.

Enzyme-rich **PINEAPPLE** will brighten your day and your skin!

CUCUMBERS are great for cooling and de-puffing. Plus, they're more than 90 percent water. Talk about hydrating!

Antioxidant-rich and potassium-packed, the humble **BANANA** may just be your beauty bestie.

Save that peel! Slice off a piece of **BANANA PEEL** and massage the inside gently over your skin for a few minutes to brighten, soften, and tone. Rinse your skin when you're done.

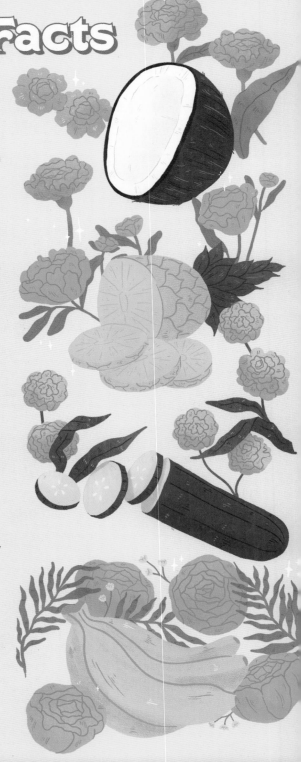

Dang! **POMEGRANATE JUICE** contains three times as many antioxidants as other fruit juices.

The probiotics, vitamins, and minerals found in fermented foods like **KEFIR** (fermented cow's milk) hydrate and moisturize your skin and may also soothe inflammatory conditions like acne and rosacea. Just stick with kefir and avoid slapping other fermented goodies like kimchi or sauerkraut on your face.

The stunning color of **BLUEBERRIES** is caused by anthocyanins, powerful antioxidants that shield your skin against the pesky free radicals (unstable atoms and molecules) out to damage your gorgeous self.

The best beauty product in your spice drawer? **TURMERIC!** It slows down skin damage, smooths texture, evens skin tone, and fights inflammation.

Naturally and gently exfoliate with **BROWN SUGAR**. It's strong enough to scrub away dry skin but gentle enough for sensitive skin.

Think **HYDRATING** and moisturizing are the same? Think again. Hydrators deliver water to the skin. Moisturizers lock it in. And, gorgeous, you need both.

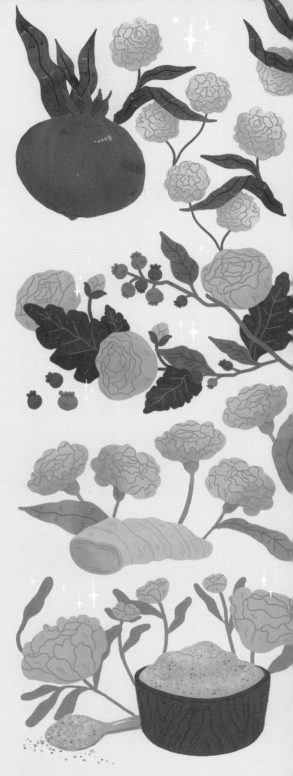

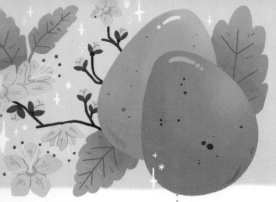

Egg on Your Face

No need to be embarrassed by excess oil and a dull complexion. Just crack open an egg and kiss your skincare worries goodbye.

INGREDIENTS

 1 egg white

 ½ cup papaya (skin peeled, seeds removed, cut into pieces, thawed if frozen)

 1 teaspoon raw honey

TOOLS

 Blender

Smoothing
Brightening
Pore-shrinking
Oil-eliminating
Breakout-busting

 1 Put all ingredients into the blender.

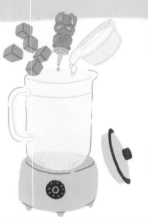

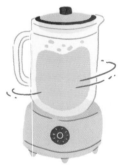 **2** Blend until the mixture is smooth.

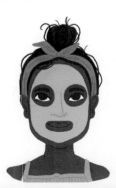 **3** Apply for 10–20 minutes, then rinse.

Let's Go Avo-Coco-Nuts

Avocado, coconut oil, and honey are a hydration triple threat. Quench thirsty skin with a dose of this restoring and energizing multi-moisturizer.

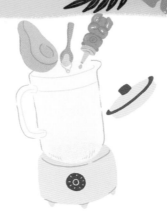

1   Put all ingredients into the blender.

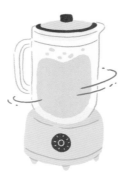

2   Blend until the mixture is smooth.

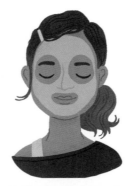

3   Apply for 10–20 minutes, then rinse.

INGREDIENTS

 ½ of one ripe avocado (skin and pit removed)

 2 tablespoons raw honey

 1 teaspoon room-temperature coconut oil

TOOLS

 Blender

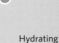

Hydrating

Smoothing

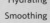

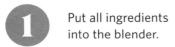
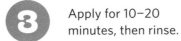

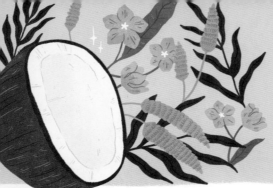

Coconut Ka-Pow!

Coconut oil penetrates deep into your skin for lasting hydration, while oats lock in moisture and clear away dead cells to give dry skin a double punch. WHAM!

INGREDIENTS

 3 tablespoons oats

 1 teaspoon room-temperature coconut oil

 2 tablespoons warm water

TOOLS

 Blender

Healing
Hydrating

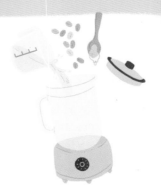

1 Put all ingredients into the blender.

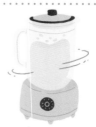

2 Blend until the mixture is a smooth paste.

3 Apply for 10–20 minutes. Remove sheet mask if using.

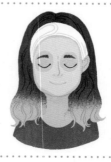

4 Gently massage your face with small, circular motions for 2 minutes, then rinse.

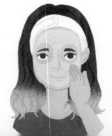

Papa-Yaaasss

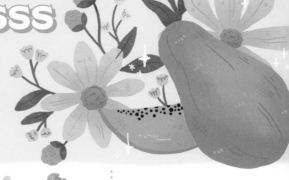

Gently exfoliate, protect, and strengthen your skin with the power of papaya. The incredibly juicy fruit contains a plethora of vitamins and minerals for smooth, glowing, and healthy skin.

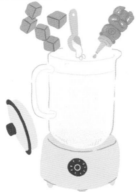

1 Put all ingredients into the blender.

INGREDIENTS

 ½ of one papaya (skin peeled, seeds removed, cut into pieces, thawed if frozen)

 2 teaspoons milk

 1 tablespoon raw honey

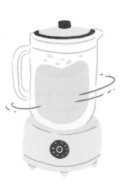

2 Blend until the mixture is smooth.

TOOLS

 Blender

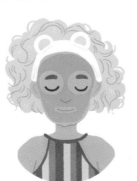

3 Apply for 10–20 minutes, then rinse.

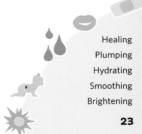

Healing
Plumping
Hydrating
Smoothing
Brightening

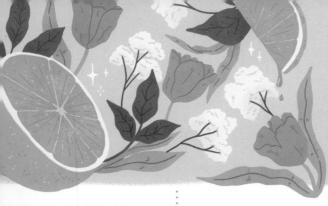

Squeeze the Day

Keep your pores clean, reduce breakouts, and repair damage with this grapefruit-and-yogurt mixture.

INGREDIENTS

 2 tablespoons grapefruit juice

 ¼ cup plain Greek yogurt

 ½ cup granulated sugar

 1 tablespoon raw honey

TOOLS

 Mixing bowl

 Spoon

Healing
Smoothing
Acne-fighting
Oil-eliminating
Breakout-busting

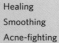
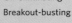
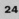

 1 Put all ingredients into the mixing bowl.

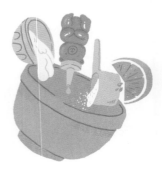

2 Mix into a smooth paste.

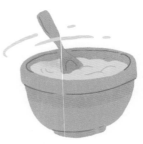

3 Apply for 10–20 minutes, then rinse.

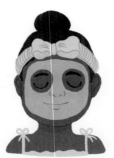

No One Stacks Up to You

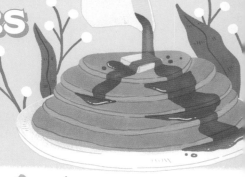

Embrace major weekend vibes with a pancake-inspired detox mask. Just skip the skillet and smooth this yummy mixture on your face for the ultimate beauty brunch.

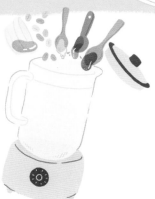

 1 Put all ingredients into the blender.

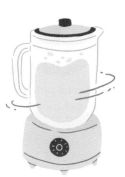 **2** Blend until the mixture is a smooth paste.

3 Apply for 10–20 minutes, then rinse.

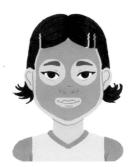

INGREDIENTS

 1 egg yolk

 ¼ cup oats

 1 teaspoon maple syrup

 1 teaspoon room-temperature coconut oil

 1 tablespoon olive oil

TOOLS

 Blender

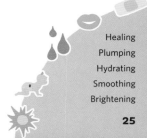

Healing
Plumping
Hydrating
Smoothing
Brightening

Season's Greetings

Open up those pores and prevent future breakouts with a jolly little moisturizing mask. Every season 'tis the season for great skin!

INGREDIENTS

 2 teaspoons ground nutmeg

 2 teaspoons ground cinnamon

 2 tablespoons raw honey

 1 teaspoon milk

TOOLS

 Blender

FYI: Nutmeg and cinnamon might cause your skin to tingle. If this feeling isn't your thing, wash off this mask ASAP.

Plumping
Hydrating
Acne-fighting
Oil-eliminating
Breakout-busting

 1 Put all ingredients into the blender.

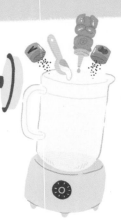

 2 Blend until the mixture is smooth.

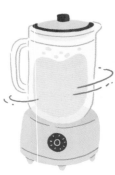

 3 Apply for 10–20 minutes, then rinse.

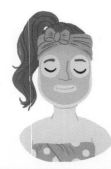

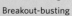

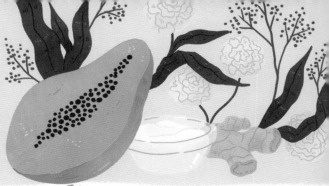

Spice Up Your Life

Whether you're feeling scary, sporty, or posh, brighten up your beauty routine with an antioxidant, antiaging, and acne-eliminating mask.

 1 Put all ingredients into the blender.

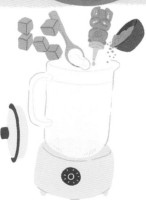

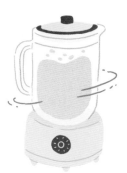 **2** Blend until the mixture is smooth.

3 Apply for 10–20 minutes, then rinse.

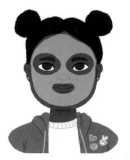

INGREDIENTS

 ½ cup papaya (skin peeled, seeds removed, cut into pieces, thawed if frozen)

 ½ teaspoon ground turmeric

 1 teaspoon raw honey

 1 teaspoon plain Greek yogurt

TOOLS

 Blender

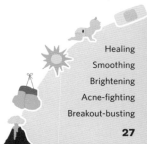
Healing
Smoothing
Brightening
Acne-fighting
Breakout-busting

Matcha Made in Heaven

Enrich and energize your look with this matcha-infused antioxidant mask. Add a dash of sandalwood to heal daily damage and that pimple you really shouldn't have popped last night.

INGREDIENTS

 1 tablespoon matcha tea

 1 teaspoon raw honey

 1 teaspoon ground cinnamon

 1 teaspoon sandalwood essential oil

TOOLS

 Mixing bowl

 Spoon

FYI: Cinnamon might cause your skin to tingle. If this feeling isn't your thing, wash off this mask ASAP.

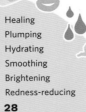

Healing
Plumping
Hydrating
Smoothing
Brightening
Redness-reducing

1 Brew the tea with one cup of water and let steep for 3 minutes. Allow the tea to cool slightly.

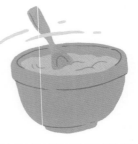

2 Put all ingredients into the mixing bowl.

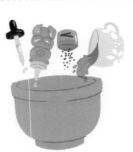

3 Mix into a smooth paste.

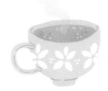

4 Apply for 10–20 minutes, then rinse.

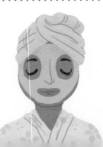

Brew-tiful Inside & Out

Use this three-ingredient fix to diminish under-eye puffiness and swelling while tightening and toning.

1
Put all ingredients into the mixing bowl.

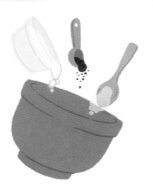

2
Mix into a smooth paste.

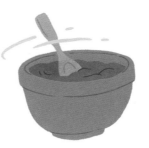

3
Apply for 10–20 minutes, then rinse.

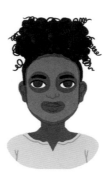

INGREDIENTS

  1 egg white

  2 teaspoons coffee grounds

  1 tablespoon room-temperature coconut oil

TOOLS

  Mixing bowl

  Spoon

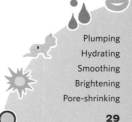

Plumping
Hydrating
Smoothing
Brightening
Pore-shrinking

Face the Facts

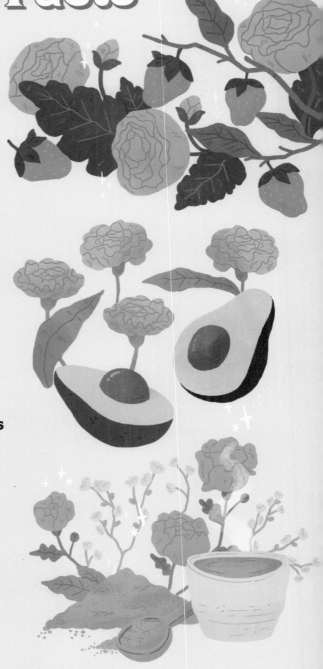

The salicylic acid (the same ingredient found in acne-fighting face washes) in **STRAWBERRIES** can dissolve oil and prevent breakouts.

Aloe isn't for everyone, and it's far from the only natural **AFTER-SUN SOLUTION**. Greek yogurt is strained more than traditional yogurt, making it thicker and packed with more probiotics. Honey has been used to treat burns since ancient Egypt. And berries protect your skin against UV radiation.

Far from being the pits, **AVOCADOS** are nutrient-dense with dozens of vitamins and minerals that are good for you—inside and out.

Your Monday morning **MATCHA** latte is absolutely antioxidant abundant, making it the perfect potion to detox and rejuvenate skin.

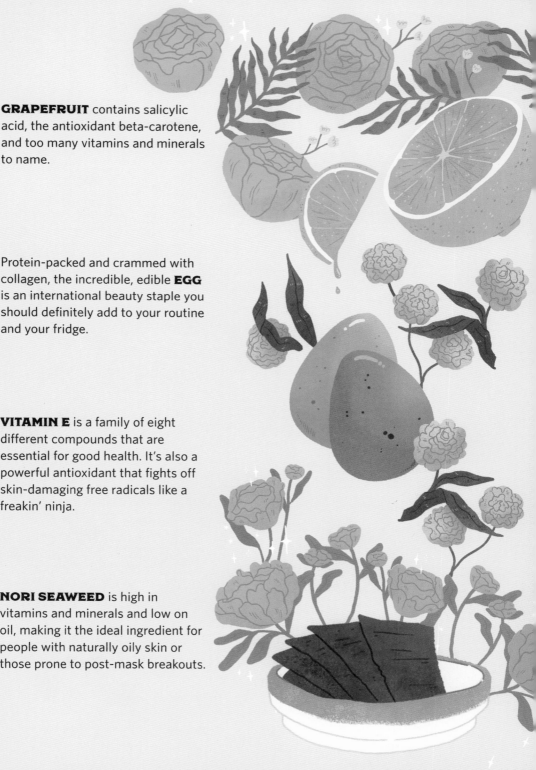

GRAPEFRUIT contains salicylic acid, the antioxidant beta-carotene, and too many vitamins and minerals to name.

Protein-packed and crammed with collagen, the incredible, edible **EGG** is an international beauty staple you should definitely add to your routine and your fridge.

VITAMIN E is a family of eight different compounds that are essential for good health. It's also a powerful antioxidant that fights off skin-damaging free radicals like a freakin' ninja.

NORI SEAWEED is high in vitamins and minerals and low on oil, making it the ideal ingredient for people with naturally oily skin or those prone to post-mask breakouts.

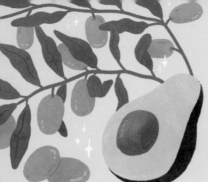

Olive Me Loves Olive You

Improve skin tone, minimize dark spots, and cleanse and condition with an enriching olive oil and avocado mask.

INGREDIENTS

 1 ripe avocado (skin and pit removed)

 2 tablespoons plain Greek yogurt

 1 tablespoon olive oil

 1 tablespoon raw honey

TOOLS

Blender

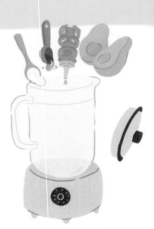

1 Put all ingredients into the blender.

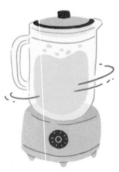

2 Blend until the mixture is smooth.

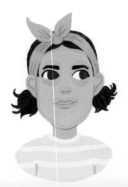

3 Apply for 10–20 minutes, then rinse.

Healing
Hydrating
Smoothing
Brightening
Redness-reducing

Aloe You Vera Much

Show your skin just how much you love it with a blend of natural ingredients that soothes sunburns and irritation.

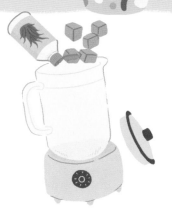

1   Put all ingredients into the blender.

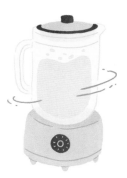

2   Blend until the mixture is smooth.

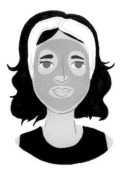

3   Apply for 10–20 minutes, then rinse.

INGREDIENTS

 ½ of one papaya (skin peeled, seeds removed, cut into pieces, thawed if frozen)

 1 tablespoon aloe vera gel

TOOLS

 Blender

Healing
Hydrating
Redness-reducing

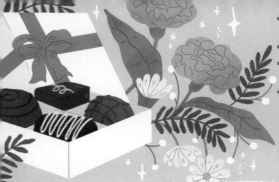

Mississippi Mud Mask

Energize and exfoliate with a decadently delicious chocolate, oat, and yogurt moisturizer.

INGREDIENTS

 4 tablespoons dark chocolate, melted

 1 tablespoon plain Greek yogurt

 2 teaspoons oats

TOOLS

Blender

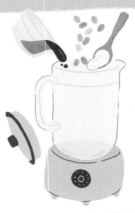

1 Put all ingredients into the blender.

2 Blend until the mixture is a smooth paste.

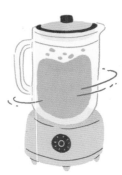

Healing
Hydrating
Smoothing
Pore-shrinking
Oil-eliminating

3 Apply for 10–20 minutes, then rinse.

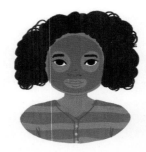

Under the Sea

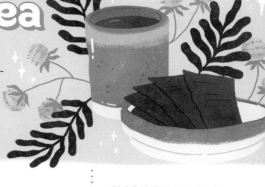

Draw out impurities with a cleansing seaweed-and-green-tea mask. Anti-inflammatory and antioxidant-packed, this purifying mixture reduces redness and keeps skin looking as fresh as the sea.

SKIP THE SHEET! This mask goes directly on your face!

INGREDIENTS

 4–6 sheets nori seaweed

 2 tablespoons freshly brewed strong green tea

TOOLS

 Bowl

1 Brew the tea with one cup of water and let steep for 3 minutes. Allow the tea to cool slightly.

2 Place the nori into the bowl.

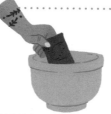

3 Pour the green tea on the sheets of nori, allowing the nori to soak for 1–2 minutes.

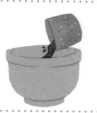

4 Remove the nori from the tea, let the excess drip off, and place the nori directly onto your face.

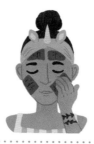

5 Apply for 10–20 minutes, then discard the used nori and rinse your skin.

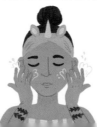

Healing
Smoothing
Brightening
Redness-reducing

35

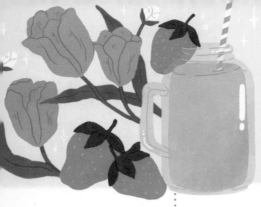

Strawberry Shake It Up

Apply this smoothie-like treat to your skin to prevent breakouts and reduce inflammation.

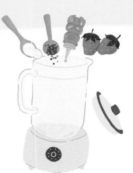

INGREDIENTS

 5 strawberries (thawed if frozen)

 4 tablespoons plain Greek yogurt

 1 tablespoon raw honey

 1 tablespoon chia seeds

TOOLS

 Blender

1 Put all ingredients into the blender.

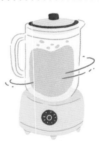

2 Blend until the mixture is smooth.

3 Apply for 10–20 minutes. Remove sheet mask if using.

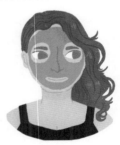

4 Gently massage your face with small, circular motions for 2 minutes, then rinse.

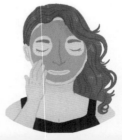

Hydrating
Brightening
Oil-eliminating
Breakout-busting
Redness-reducing

Bananarama

Oats and banana are one delicious combination for an extraordinary exfoliating experience. The addition of raw honey hydrates and softens.

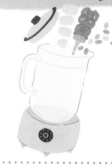

1. Put all ingredients into the blender.

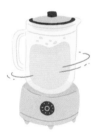

2. Blend until the mixture is a smooth paste.

3. Apply for 10–20 minutes. Remove sheet mask if using.

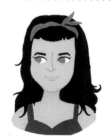

4. Gently massage your face with small, circular motions for 2 minutes, then rinse.

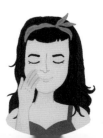

INGREDIENTS

  ½ of one banana

2 tablespoons oats

  2 tablespoons raw honey

TOOLS

Blender

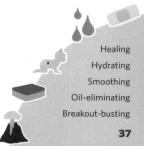

Healing
Hydrating
Smoothing
Oil-eliminating
Breakout-busting

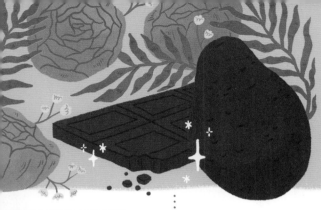

Bravo-Cado!

Plump things up with a cocoa powder and avocado concoction for standing ovation–worthy skin.

INGREDIENTS

 ½ of one ripe avocado (skin and pit removed)

 1 tablespoon cocoa powder

 1 teaspoon plain Greek yogurt

 1 teaspoon raw honey

TOOLS

 Blender

 Plumping
 Hydrating
Smoothing
Brightening

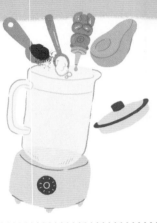

1 Put all ingredients into the blender.

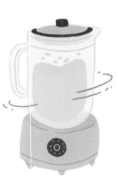

2 Blend until the mixture is smooth.

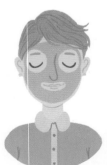

3 Apply for 10–20 minutes, then rinse.

Feeling Grapeful

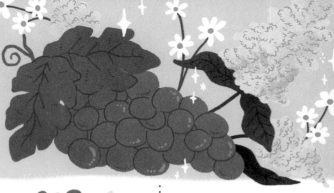

No matter what state your skin is in, anyone can benefit from this anti-inflammatory, brightening, and acne-fighting mask.

1   Put all ingredients into the blender.

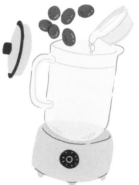

INGREDIENTS

 6–7 grapes

 1 egg white

TOOLS

 Blender

2   Blend until the mixture is smooth.

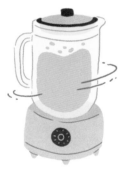

3   Apply for 10–20 minutes, then rinse.

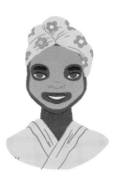

Healing
Smoothing
Brightening
Acne-fighting
Redness-reducing

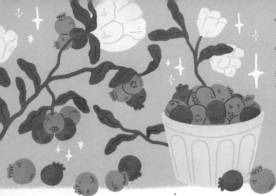

Berry Cute Skin

Brighten, plump, and protect your skin from gross pollutants with vitamins B and C, found in supercute and super-good-for-you cranberries.

INGREDIENTS

 8–10 cranberries (thawed if frozen)

3 tablespoons plain Greek yogurt (or as needed)

 2 teaspoons raw honey

TOOLS

Blender

Plumping
Hydrating
Brightening

 1 Put all ingredients into the blender.

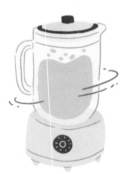

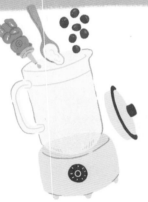

2 Blend until the mixture is a smooth paste.

3 Apply for 10–20 minutes, then rinse.

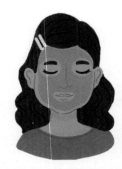

Honey Bun

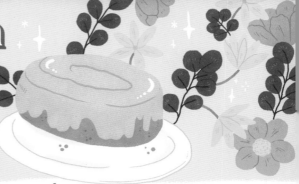

Soften up and cool down with a honey-soaked moisturizing mask. The addition of baking soda makes it a lovely anti-inflammatory and antibacterial as well.

1 Put all ingredients into the mixing bowl.

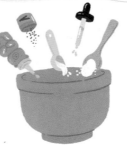

2 Mix into a smooth paste.

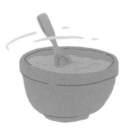

3 Apply for 10–20 minutes. Remove sheet mask if using.

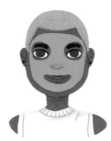

4 Gently massage your face with small, circular motions for another 2 minutes, then rinse.

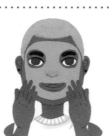

INGREDIENTS

 3 tablespoons baking soda

 3 teaspoons milk

 1 teaspoon raw honey

 1 teaspoon vitamin E oil

 ¼ teaspoon ground cinnamon

TOOLS

 Mixing bowl

 Spoon

FYI: Cinnamon might cause your skin to tingle. If this feeling isn't your thing, wash off this mask ASAP.

First time using baking soda for skincare? Test this mixture on the inside of your wrist beforehand.

Healing
Hydrating
Acne-fighting
Oil-eliminating
Breakout-busting
Redness-reducing

41

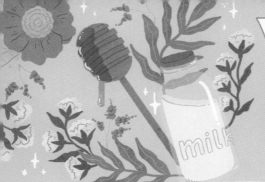

Wholey Cow

Follow in the footsteps of Cleopatra, who famously bathed in oats, milk, and honey. The lactic acid found in milk naturally eats away at dead skin, the antibacterial properties of raw honey clear away acne and dirt, and the oats scrub and soothe.

INGREDIENTS

 3 tablespoons oats

 1 tablespoon milk

 1 tablespoon raw honey

TOOLS

 Blender

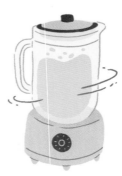

1 Put all ingredients into the blender.

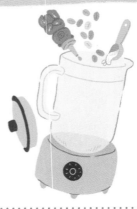

2 Blend until the mixture is a smooth paste.

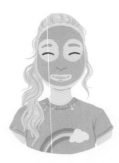

3 Apply for 10–20 minutes, then rinse.

Brightening
Acne-fighting
Pore-shrinking
Oil-eliminating
Breakout-busting

Oat-Em-Gee

It's tea time! Put the kettle on and say buh-bye to dry, itchy, rough skin with this gentle brew of oats, green tea, and honey.

1 Brew the tea with one cup of water and let steep for 3 minutes. Allow the tea to cool slightly.

2 Put all ingredients into the blender.

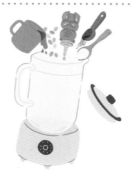

3 Blend until the mixture is a smooth paste.

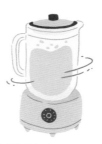

4 Apply for 10–20 minutes, then rinse.

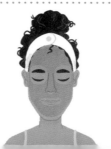

INGREDIENTS

 3 tablespoons freshly brewed strong green tea

 1 ½ tablespoons oats

 1 teaspoon raw honey

 1 tablespoon apple cider vinegar

 2 tablespoons plain Greek yogurt

TOOLS

Blender

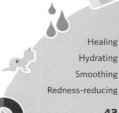

Healing
Hydrating
Smoothing
Redness-reducing

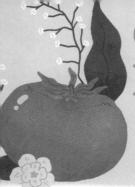

Gorgeous from My Head To-Ma-Toes

Keep sun damage and premature aging at bay while retaining smooth and supple skin—all thanks to the powerful antioxidant lycopene, the natural pigment that makes tomatoes red.

INGREDIENTS

 2 tablespoons aloe vera gel

 1 tablespoon tomato juice

 1 tablespoon pumpkin puree

TOOLS

 Mixing bowl

 Spoon

Healing
Plumping
Smoothing
Breakout-busting

 1 Put all ingredients into the mixing bowl.

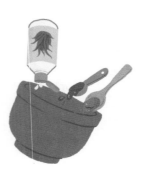

 2 Mix until smooth.

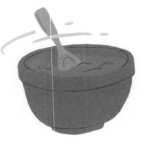

 3 Apply for 10–20 minutes, then rinse.

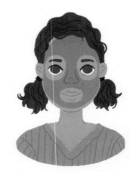

44

Cool as a Cute-cumber

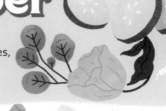

Feeling frazzled? Give your skin a chill pill and cover it in rich antioxidants, anti-inflammatories, and essential vitamins like A, B, C, biotin, and potassium.

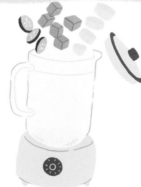

1 Put all ingredients into the blender.

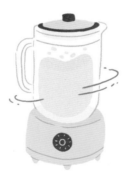

2 Blend until the mixture is smooth.

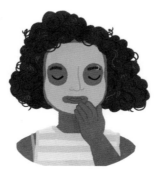

3 Apply for 10–20 minutes, then rinse.

INGREDIENTS

½ of one cucumber (cut into slices)

¼ cup papaya (skin peeled, seeds removed, cut into pieces, thawed if frozen)

½ of one banana

TOOLS

Blender

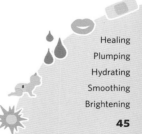

Healing
Plumping
Hydrating
Smoothing
Brightening

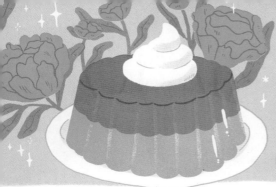

You Had Me at Jell-O

This mask works double duty: tightening and toning your skin while also drying and cleaning out clogged pores. Show me the honey!

SKIP THE SHEET! This mask goes directly on your face!

INGREDIENTS

 1 ½ tablespoons milk

 1 tablespoon unflavored gelatin

 1 tablespoon raw honey

TOOLS

 Microwave-safe mixing bowl

 Spoon

 Microwave

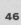 Healing
Pore-shrinking
Oil-eliminating
Breakout-busting

1 Combine all ingredients in the microwave-safe mixing bowl.

2 Microwave for 30 seconds.

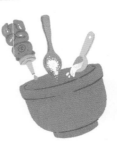

3 Mix into a smooth paste, allowing the mixture to cool if hot.

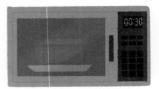

4 Apply evenly in a thin layer for 10–20 minutes, then rinse.

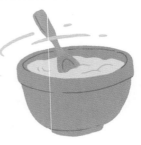

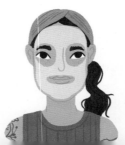

Guac My World

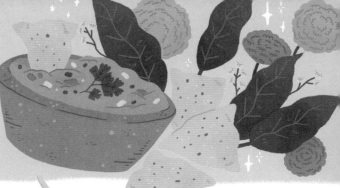

Tortilla chips and toast aren't the only things you should be covering with avocado. Slather on this spread to prevent puffiness and redness.

1 Put all ingredients into the blender.

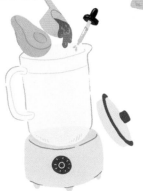

INGREDIENTS

 ½ of one ripe avocado (skin and pit removed)

 1 teaspoon vitamin E oil

 Splash of carrot juice (optional)

2 Blend until the mixture is smooth.

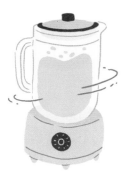

TOOLS

 Blender

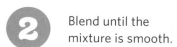

3 Apply for 10–20 minutes, then rinse.

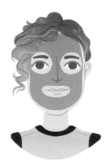

Healing
Plumping
Hydrating
Smoothing
Redness-reducing

Odd Dot
An imprint of Macmillan Publishing Group, LLC
120 Broadway, New York, NY 10271
OddDot.com

Text Copyright © 2019 by Odd Dot
Illustrations Copyright © 2019 by Emma Trithart

Library of Congress Cataloging-in-Publication Data is available.
ISBN 978-1-250-20812-5

EDITOR
Justin Krasner

COVER AND INTERIOR DESIGNER
Carolyn Bahar

ILLUSTRATOR
Emma Trithart

Our books may be purchased in bulk for promotional, educational, or business use. Please contact your local bookseller or the Macmillan Corporate and Premium Sales Department at (800) 221-7945 ext. 5442 or by email at MacmillanSpecialMarkets@macmillan.com.

Printed in China in September 2019 by Hung Hing Off-set Printing Co., Ltd.,
Heshan City, Guangdong Province
First edition, 2019

1 3 5 7 9 10 8 6 4 2

DISCLAIMER: The mask mixtures in this book are for external use only. Avoid contact with eyes. In the event of eye contact, rinse immediately with water. Avoid using on skin that is sensitive to bandages, tapes, or peel-off masks. This book is for entertainment purposes only and does not provide medical advice.

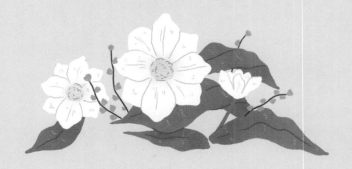